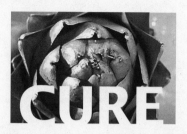

Indigestion, Heartburn, Cholesterol, Triglyceride and Liver Problems with

Artichoke Extract

by
Gary Ross, M.D.
and
David Steinman

Disclaimer: The material in this presentation is for informational
purposes only and not intended for the treatment or diagnosis of
individual disease. Please, visit a qualified medical or other health
professional for specifically diagnosing any ailments mentioned or
discussed in detail in this material.

This information is presented by independent medical experts
whose sources of information include scientific studies from the
world's medical and scientific literature, doctors' patient and
other clinical and anecdotal reports.

ISBN 1-893910-01-6

First Printing, March 1999.

Published by Freedom Press
1801 Chart Trail
Topanga, CA 90290

Bulk Orders Available: (310) 455-2995
E-mail: sales@freedompressonline.com

ET

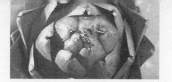

Table of Contents

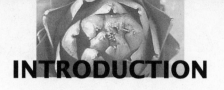

INTRODUCTION

Artichoke Extract for Indigestion, Cholesterol, Triglyceride and Liver Problems

D*o you suffer frequently from indigestion? Do you common-ly feel nausea or bloated after eating? Do you have a ten-dency to belch or suffer from flatulence after a big meal or meal rich in saturated fats? Are you sick and tired of feeling loggy after meals? Are you sick and tired of the prescription and over-the-counter antacid drugs with their own dangerous complications that your doctor prescribes and that offer only temporary relief? Don't despair. There is help.*

Indigestion may be the most prevalent complaint people have, outside the common cold. In fact, estimates are that about 30 percent of people today suffer from chronic indigestion. Technically, this condition is known as dyspepsia. Its symptoms are not only personally uncomfortable, they may be socially embarrassing! A related complication of indigestion includes acid reflux.

Considering our modern diet and the industrial sized meal portions we often consume, loaded with saturated fat or other foods with their own difficult to digest nutrients, it's little wonder that almost everyone suffers from indigestion and related problems at one time or another. The stomach does some amazing things to its contents, grinding foods like a grist mill and releasing an acid so powerful it could burn the skin, and then assimilating nutrients into the body's tissues as well as transporting away the waste. But as we age, our ability to digest certain types of foods such as fats and carbohydrates often becomes impaired.

Indigestion (also known as dyspepsia) and related conditions such as irritable bowel disease may be the most prevalent complaints people have today, outside of the common cold. In fact, estimates are that about 30 percent of people today suffer from some form of chronic indigestion. This condition can be brought on or exacerbated by use of medical drugs.

Yet, contrary to what your doctor or pharmaceutical advertising may say, one of the best cures for indigestion isn't a drug at all! It's the highly concentrated and totally safe extract of a commonly consumed vegetable: artichoke extract.

HAS YOUR DOCTOR TOLD YOU THAT YOU HAVE HIGH cholesterol or triglycerides? Do you suffer from coronary artery disease? And are you at risk for plaque or other types of coronary artery blockage?

If so, artichoke extract has shown promising evidence of gently and safely lowering cholesterol and triglycerides.

HAVE YOU EVER SUFFERED FROM LIVER DISEASE SUCH as hepatitis? Do you consume alcohol on a regular basis? Are you concerned that your liver cannot handle the ethanol overload? How about your use of over-the-counter or prescription drugs, even seemingly safe preparations such as acetaminophen (Tylenol)? Do you take these on a regular basis for your aches and pains, arthritis or other chronic conditions? If so, these could be adversely affecting your liver. Did you know that artichoke extract may be an important way of protecting your liver from these harmful effects?

The good news is that artichoke extract can protect your liver and even help to regenerate healthy cells in already-damaged liver tissues.

A CLEAR DIRECTION

Like a lot of health-conscious consumers today, you've probably heard a great deal of discussion both in the news media and among your friends about alternative medicine and especially various herbs and nutrients that may be of benefit to people suffering specific conditions. But, like many consumers today, you probably feel overwhelmed by the wide variety of natural healing agents available. And you may wonder which herbs and nutrients are proven to offer significant, medically validated health benefits—and which are safe for use. Also, you may wonder how herbs and nutrients compare to the medical drugs that your doctor typically prescribes.

Artichoke extract is one of the most well-studied natural medicines today—and one that both of us believe will become one of the important natural medicines of the new millennium. In this book, we will detail the many documented benefits of artichoke extract for conditions such as indigestion, high cholesterol and triglycerides, and liver disease, as well as compare its benefits and safety record with prescription or over-the-counter drugs that you doctor may recommend for the same conditions. You'll be amazed at how beneficial artichoke extract has been proved to be, and you'll be delighted with its proven safety record.

Gary Ross, M.D., and David Steinman
March 1999

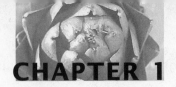

Artichoke Extract—
Natural Medicine with
Diverse Benefits

Indigestion? High cholesterol or triglycerides? Poor liver function? If any of these diseases or health conditions are a concern of yours, artichoke extract, a widely popular medicine in Germany but virtually unknown in the United States, may be one of the most important supplements for your daily health program.

You've probably heard of artichokes and have even consumed them. Like most vegetables, artichokes are good for us. But the active ingredients of this tall, composite herb with its spiked green flower are even better for our health than we may realize. Also known as the globe artichoke (or *Cynara scolymus* in Latin), this thistle-like plant is a member of the compositae family which includes the aster, daisy, dandelion, marigold, sunflower, thistle and zinnia.

You may never have known that a highly concentrated form of artichoke extract is actually a many-talented, yet little-known, natural medicine that is certain to take its place in the new millennium as one of the most important dietary supplements available to the American public.

But what exactly is artichoke extract? Is it safe? What benefits can you expect? Could its powers be so great as to replace your prescription or over-the-counter (OTC) drugs? This chapter will provide you with an overview of the powers of artichoke extract to help to improve your health.

There are many reasons why you should consider adding artichoke extract to your daily health program.

◆ Do you suffer from bloating, gas and other symptoms of indigestion after eating meals?
◆ Are you one of the millions of Americans with high cholesterol?
◆ Has anyone in your family been stricken with a heart attack, stroke, or cancer?
◆ Do you live in an urban setting where environmental pollution is prevalent?
◆ Do you regularly consume alcohol or work in an occupation where you are regularly exposed to chemical toxins?

If you answered *yes* to any of these questions, then artichoke extract is an important supplement for you to use on a daily basis.

In each of these cases, artichoke extract can help to provide you with an edge to overcome these health threats and perhaps extend both your overall life span and your healthy living span by several years or more.

You might be wondering if you couldn't just consume more artichokes at dinner. Unfortunately, beyond the familiar artichoke heart and the rubbery blossom leaves, what's most beneficial are properties derived from parts of the plant that never reach the dinner table—the thistle-like leaves along the base of its stem. So chances are consuming artichoke even regularly at dinnertime will not provide consumers with the concentrated benefits to be derived from using artichoke extract as a dietary supplement.

HISTORY OF MEDICINAL USES

The basal leaves of this plant have been used as a medicinal agent since the fourth century BC. Artichoke extract was a favorite medicine of the Middle Ages as doctors first began to recognize that the body's liver influences so many parameters of human health.

Since that time, artichoke leaf extract's health benefits have been recognized the world over. The French have long advocated artichoke juice for its use as a liver tonic, and scientists from

Japan to Switzerland have noted the herb's abilities to break down fat and improve bile flow. Now, the time has come for Americans to discover the medically proven benefits of artichoke extract.

BENEFICIAL ACTIVE INGREDIENTS

According to German scientists, artichoke extract leaves contain high amounts of caffeic acid, chlorogenic acid, and mono- and di-caffeoylquinic acid derivatives such as cynarin, luteolin, luteolinglucosides, scolymoside and cynaroside. It is this extended family of caffeoylquinic acids, known generally as cynarins, which offers powerful nutritional support for the liver.

CONDITIONS ARTICHOKE EXTRACT BENEFITS

This versatile natural medicine has been shown to help with nausea, indigestion, gallbladder and biliary problems, liver congestion and other liver problems, high blood lipids and diabetes mellitus. The documentation on its benefits to the liver are extensive. Indeed, scientists believe that virtually all of the healthy attributes of artichoke extract, ultimately, are the result of its highly beneficial effect on liver function.

HIGHLY RESEARCHED HERB

The research on artichoke extract is quite extensive, dating all the way back to the Middle Ages. Most recently, German scientists have used modern medical and scientific techniques, including clinical studies, to not only determine whether artichoke extract delivers important health benefits and the mechanism of action for these benefits, but also its metabolic and pharmacologic pathways within the human body.

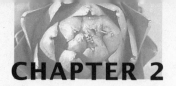

CHAPTER 2

Artichoke Extract
for Indigestion

Fed up with chronic gas, nausea, belching, bloating and even vomiting? Ask your doctor for help and he or she will probably respond by first taking your history and performing a physical examination. Your doctor will feel the esophagus and check for any types of perforations as well as test you for the presence of the ulcer-causing bacteria, *Helicobacter pylori*. If the finding for *H. pylori* is positive, the patient will be treated with drugs such as omeprazole (Prilosec), Pepto-Bismol, and various antibiotics. If the findings for *H. pylori* are negative, the doctor usually writes out a prescription for a drug that will relieve symptoms temporarily by interfering with the natural digestion process and blocking the body's acid secretions, or by telling the patient to simply take more Tums or another OTC antacid.

If the doctor is still not sure what's causing a patient's indigestion, the patient may be given an upper gastrointestinal tract X-ray or the doctor may use an endoscope to rule out stomach cancer.

Very often, however, these quick fixes offer no permanent solution. The problem is that the next time you eat you will once again end up suffering from uncomfortable, sometimes embarrassing symptoms of indigestion.

Using typical prescription or over the counter drugs offers a temporary fix but doesn't attack your problem at the source.

Your doctor has treated your symptoms but without initiating the healing process within. The real solution to indigestion is to understand the cause and attack the problem at its root.

What's more, some such drugs for indigestion may be cancer-causing or disturb hormonal balances in men and women (see pages 16-17).

When more serious illnesses are ruled out, doctors practicing complementary medicine prefer to treat their patients with nat-

What is Indigestion?

If you feel gaseous or bloated, suffer excessive flatulence, constipation, nausea or even must vomit after meals on a regular basis, then you may be suffering from chronic indigestion. Known medically as dyspepsia, indigestion is characterized by upper abdominal discomfort and pain with bloating and fullness after eating. Other symptoms can include belching, bloating, burping, heartburn, loss of appetite, regurgitation, early feeling of fullness, perhaps even nausea and vomiting. The symptoms typically occur one to two hours after a meal and may be temporarily improved by taking antacids. About one-third of Americans today suffer from chronic indigestion.

Mild, occasional indigestion is generally transient and self-limiting without the need of medical care. But when indigestion becomes a chronic problem that accompanies practically every meal, then you have a serious problem. Often overlooked by the medical profession is that a significant cause of indigestion is *not* necessarily oversecretion of hydrochloric acid but the result of poor liver function—particularly what medical experts call congested liver where bile flow is inhibited.

This liver disorder, which is also called cholestasis (lack of bile flow), impairs the body's ability to properly digest and utilize the foods which you take in. This may lead to constipation and the other symptoms of indigestion. Poor bile flow often leads to intolerance of fat and, thus, dyspepsia or indigestion.

ural therapies such as dietary changes and nutritional supplements. Still, indigestion is a difficult condition to get rid of and doctors are always looking for new natural approaches to addressing this problem. That is why we believe, although still new to most doctors in the United States, artichoke extract is going to soon be recognized as a welcome addition to medical practice. Along with the Hippocratic Oath, "Do no harm," artichoke extract is safe and worth a try to help people who are suffering indigestion. It's a different way of looking at helping persons with indigestion but definitely a viable way of addressing the problem. Artichoke extract is a natural cure that will in fact attack your indigestion problem at its source.

HOW ARTICHOKE EXTRACT WORKS

An often overlooked key to optimal digestion is healthy bile flow. Artichoke extract is one of the few known safe substances today that actually stimulates the liver's bile flow. Bile is a viscid, alkaline, yellowish-green fluid excreted from the liver, stored in the gallbladder, and released into the intestine to aid in the digestion and absorption of fats. Bile contains more than 97 percent water. Its most important components are bile salts including bile acids, cholesterol, lecithin, cations (Na, K, and Ca) and anions such as chloride and bicarbonate.

Bile acids are natural detergents. They induce bile flow and liquefy fats that the body takes in. Bile also plays an important role in softening the stool by promoting the incorporation of water. Without enough bile, the stool can become quite hard and difficult to pass. Bile also helps to keep the small intestine free from microorganisms (parasites).

Disturbances of the liver's bile flow often lead to intolerance of fat and dyspepsia. Today, especially among European doctors, it is increasingly recognized that an increase in bile secretion is regarded as an essential and effective principle in the treatment of indigestion. Both experimental and clinical human studies have shown that indigestion is rooted, at least partly, in gastric

Causes of Cholestasis

◆ Presence of gallstones
◆ Alcohol
◆ Endotoxins
◆ Hereditary disorders such as Gilbert's syndrome
◆ Hyperthyroidism or thyroxine supplementation
◆ Viral hepatitis
◆ Pregnancy

◆ Certain chemicals or drugs:
  - Natural and synthetic steroidal hormones
  - Anabolic steroids
  - Estrogens
  - Oral contraceptives
  - Aminosalicylic acid
  - Chlorothiazide
  - Erythromycin estolate
  - Mepazine
  - Phenylbutazone
  - Sulphadiazine
  - Thiouracil

Natural Medicine Journal, 1998; 1(7): 22-24.

and bile flow disorders. Increased choleresis (or optimal flow of bile) can lead to improved intestinal motility and a higher activity of fat digestion.

In today's view, the active principle of choleretically active natural medicines such as artichoke extract is therefore seen as beneficial both in secretory support of the digestive activity and in the influence on intestinal motility. However, only a very few preparations have a proven choleretic effect. Artichoke extract is one of these.

WHAT IF THE DOCTOR SAYS TO USE A PRESCRIPTION OR OTC DRUG FOR CHRONIC INDIGESTION?

It is true that most doctors typically prescribe drugs that inhibit gastric acid secretions or that stimulate gastric emptying of solids and liquids, and that these can temporarily effectively alleviate your symptoms. However, unless your condition is life-threatening (chances are, it isn't), there is no need to start with medically prescribed or over-the-counter drugs. It would be far smarter to use the gentle yet effective healing powers of a safe and natural medicine such as artichoke extract. As you can see from Table 2.1 (page 16), typically prescribed medical drugs are not without complications, some of which can be quite serious.

Most typically, doctors recommend drugs known as H2 receptor antagonists like cimetidine (Tagamet®), famotidine (Pepcid®), nazatidine, and ranitidine (Zantac®). These drugs which are available over-the-counter work by occupying sites on the surface of gastric cells. These sites are called histamine H2 receptors. When specific types of histamines (a type of substance composed from ammonia) attach to them, these receptors signal the stomach cells to secrete various chemicals such as hydrochloric acid that help to digest food. By taking up residence on these receptors, such drugs prevent histamines from occupying the spaces on these receptors and stimulating the secretory activity of the cells. The volume of acidic secretions in the stomach is, therefore, reduced. This temporarily reduces your symptoms. But this is only a temporary solution, since excess acid secretions often are not the cause of indigestion but merely a symptom.

Drugs such as antacids (Mylanta, Maalox, or Tums) can help to neutralize stomach acidity by adding a buffering mineral such as calcium.

Work with Your Doctor to Rule-out Other More Serious Causes of Indigestion

Occasionally, indigestion can be a symptom of another, more serious problem. For this reason, you should see your doctor for a thorough check-up. Chronic indigestion may also be associated with conditions such as Crohn's disease; colon cancer; inadequate or excess stomach acid; inflammatory conditions of the stomach or pancreas; ulcers; scleroderma; lupus; parasites or amoebae; even a weak heart; or diabetes.

Table 2.1

SAFE SHOPPER'S CHART

Artichoke Extract vs. Medical Drugs for Indigestion

Typically Prescribed Drug or Natural Formula	Adverse Reactions/ Possible Chronic Toxicity
Artichoke Extract	None.
Magnesium hydroxide (Maalox, Milk of Magnesia, Mylanta, Tums)	No significant adverse or chronic effects. Possible drug interactions. Avoid products that list aluminum compounds as ingredients.
Cimetidine (Tagamet)	Headaches, gynecomastia, impotence, decreased white blood cell counts, congested liver, increases in plasma creatinine, experimental evidence of possible carcinogenic effect.
Cisapride (Propulsid®)	Headaches, diarrhea, abdominal pain, dyspepsia, urinary tract infection, increased frequency of urination, abnormal vision.
Famotidine (Pepcid)	Headaches, dizziness, constipation, diarrhea. Possibly arrhythmia, palpitations, tinnitus.
Metoclopramide (Reglan®)	Restlessness, drowsiness, fatigue and lassitude, depression, dystonia, tardive dyskinesia, elevated prolactin (possibly increased cancer risk), gynecomastia, impotence.
Omeprazole (Prilosec®)	Abdominal pain, diarrhea, headaches, possible carcinogenicity based on experimental studies.
Ranitidine (Zantac)	Severe headaches, dizziness, insomnia, vertigo, arrhythmia, constipation, diarrhea, nausea, increases in liver SGPT values, blood count changes.

Motility enhancement drugs are also used. These include cisapride (Propulsid®) or metoclopramide (Reglan®). These work by stimulating gastric emptying of both solids and liquids.

PRESCRIPTION AND OTC DRUG COMPLICATIONS

Although prescription or OTC drugs' side effects or complications are often only mild, occasionally they may be quite serious in some patients. For example, people using famotidine or ranitidine may be more likely to suffer from mild to severe headaches, dizziness, constipation, or diarrhea.

The complications from cimetidine may be more serious. While not cancer-causing in rodents, cimetidine does alter the body's metabolism of estrogen, causing gynecomastia in men.[1] These estrogenic effects are consistent with a single report of breast cancer in a man who had been treated with cimetidine.[2] "After being on [the drug] for eight months . . . he was found to have a hard malignant mass replacing his right breast." Clearly, human studies on this drug are overdue, especially as it is in very common use.

The *Physicians' Desk Reference* warns that serious heart arrhythmias have been reported in patients who are using cisapride with other medications, including some common antibiotics. The drug could potentially impair fertility, according to experimental studies.

Metoclopramide can cause mental depression including suicidal tendencies, Parkinsonian-like symptoms, and tardive dyskinesia; other complications include restlessness, drowsiness, fatigue and lassitude; levels of the hormone prolactin may be increased which can increase women's risk for breast cancer.

As for omeprazole (Prilosec), it may be carcinogenic, based on experimental data reported in the 1997 *Physicians' Desk Reference*. In two 24-month carcinogenicity studies in rats, omeprazole at daily doses approximately four to three-hundred-fifty-two times the human dose produced gastric ECL cell carcinoids in a dose-related manner in both male and female rats; the incidence of this effect was markedly higher in female rats, which had higher blood levels of omeprazole. Gastric carcinoids seldom occur in the untreated rat. In addition, ECL cell hyperplasia was present in all treated groups of both sexes. An unusual primary malignant tumor in the stomach was seen in one rat. No similar tumor was seen in male or female rats treated for two years. For this strain of rat no similar tumor has been noted historically, but a finding involving only one tumor is difficult to interpret. A 78-week mouse carcinogenicity study of omeprazole did not show increased tumor occurrence, but the study was not conclusive.

For a complete break-out of the safety of commonly pre-scribed drugs for indigestion, see Table 2.1 (page 16).

NATURAL MEDICINE—THE BETTER CHOICE

What is the difference between *treatment* and *healing*? This is a key question for anyone who truly desires great health. Treatment, in the narrowest sense, is the application of drugs or surgery, the bringing into play of some foreign object, often alien to the body's natural ecology, to stop illness' symp-toms—but from the outside, usually not getting at the root of the problem.

Of course, emergencies, such as bacterial pneumonia, require acute *treatment*. For the lengthening "marathon" of life today, however, we want to focus our attention on promoting healing. Healing stimulates the body's own natural powers and promotes a longer and healthier life. Your body, when all is said and done, is the greatest healing pharmacy. Turning on the healing powers of your own body is key to health.

Powerful synthetic drugs have their place in medicine, par-ticularly in emergency room practice and other life-threatening situations, but for simple indigestion you will be better off work-ing with a natural medicine that is completely safe and that ini-tiates the healing process within.

Abnormalities such as prolonged gastric (stomach) emptying time or flatulence are symptoms, not the cause, of chronic indigestion.

Artichoke extract relieves symptoms by enhancing bile flow and turning on the body's own innate healing powers. Scientific studies back up its benefits.

Medical Validation

◆ As early as 1974, it was shown that artichoke preparations could increase choleresis (bile flow) in humans.[3]

◆ These results were confirmed in a second study conducted in 1992 involving 403 patients with functional disturbances of the bile duct. Some 78 percent of patients and 87 percent of the doctors who evaluated their treatment with artichoke extract rated the medicine as having "very good" effects.[4]

◆ In a 1993 study, it was shown that persons receiving artichoke extract showed a significantly higher increase in their average bile secretion when compared to persons receiving a placebo (dummy pill).[5] In this study, twenty volunteers were given either artichoke extract or a placebo and increases in their bile volume were measured after 30 and 60 minutes. The bile secretions of persons receiving the artichoke leaf extract increased an average of 127.3 percent after only 30 minutes and 151.3 percent after one hour. In contrast, the highest measured volume of bile secretion among persons receiving only placebo was a mere 39.5 percent. The higher volumes were also present up to 2½ hours later when compared to the group receiving the placebo. The researchers learned that the effects of artichoke extract occur within 30 minutes and continue for the next two hours. The researchers concluded, "It currently seems that the traditional physiotherapy of gastrointestinal disorders [with artichoke leaf extract] will once again find its deserved therapeutic rank."

◆ In a 1996 study, artichoke leaf extract was studied in a six-week surveillance study in 553 patients with non-specific digestive disorders, particularly dyspeptic discomforts and functional bile duct discomfort with which they had been suffering an average of three years prior to the study.[6] Their average age was 54.7 years. Average length of use was 43.5 days. Striking results were found among persons suffering from the most extreme symptoms. Showing improvement were: some 88 percent of patients suffering from vomiting syndrome; 82 percent with nausea; 76 percent with abdominal pain; 72 percent with loss of appetite; 71 percent with constipation; 68 percent with flatulence; and 59 percent with fat intolerance. The physicians judged the benefits to be derived from artichoke leaf extract as good to excellent in 85 percent of patients. The researchers concluded, "The results of the . . . study . . . confirm the therapeutic efficacy and high application safety [of artichoke leaf extract] with non-specific digestive disorders."

EFFICACY OF ARTICHOKE EXTRACT COMPARED TO TYPICALLY RECOMMENDED DRUGS

No comparison studies have yet been reported comparing artichoke leaf extract to commonly prescribed or over-the-counter medications. However, clinical results indicate that most patients do very well on artichoke leaf extract and that they are relieved of both their symptoms and any anxiety that they may feel having to rely for an extended duration of time on a medical drug with potentially serious complications.

WHAT ELSE CAN BE DONE TO MINIMIZE SYMPTOMS OF CHRONIC INDIGESTION?

◆ Avoid foods and medication that can aggravate your symptoms. This would include hot or spicy foods, anti-inflammatory drugs such as aspirin, ibuprofen or naproxen, and steroid medications.

◆ If you smoke, chew tobacco, or use nicotine chewing gum, quit. Smoking is an important cause of dyspepsia and slows the healing of ulcers. Your healthcare provider can give you information about quitting.

◆ Drink less alcohol, coffee (both caffeinated and "decaf"), black tea, and caffeinated soft drinks. These can irritate the stomach.
◆ Take it easy. If emotional stress contributes to your symptoms, try to identify and control sources of stress in your life.

BOTTOM LINE

You no longer need to rely solely on medical drugs for help with your indigestion problems. Artichoke extract is on its way to becoming a front-line natural medicine for the entire indigestion complex (known as dyspepsia). Its clinical validation is solid and safety assured. If you are already using medication for indigestion, consider using artichoke extract and working with your doctor or qualified health professional to reduce your medication's dosage.

Artichoke extract may be combined with other natural medicines that also can help to relieve acid indigestion, heartburn and sour or upset stomach, such as deglycyrrhizinated licorice (DGL) for overall healing of the stomach lining and acid-neutralizing calcium carbonate.

See pages 34-37 for information on how to select a quality artichoke extract formula and page 38 for information on where to obtain both our recommended artichoke extract and DGL/calcium carbonate formulas.

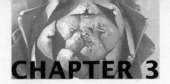

CHAPTER 3

Artichoke Extract
for Lowering Cholesterol
and Triglycerides

High levels of cholesterol and triglycerides are both indicators of increased risk for heart disease. Unfortunately, millions of Americans suffer from high blood levels of each. While medical drugs may help to reduce cholesterol and triglyceride levels, their complications may make them less desirable than a safe natural medicine such as artichoke extract.

CHOLESTEROL

Health-conscious people recognize that high levels of cholesterol in their blood increase their risk of heart disease. Cholesterol is not a fat but it is closely related to fat. It is a chemical that is an essential component in the structure of cells and is also involved in the formation of important hormones. If your diet contained no cholesterol your liver would still produce all the cholesterol you need.

However, high levels of a particular kind of cholesterol called low density lipoprotein (LDL or "bad" cholesterol) can contribute to coronary artery disease in which the blood vessels are narrowed by deposits of fatty tissues called atheromas, which are made up largely of cholesterol. Narrowing of the heart's coronary arteries by patches of atheromas can cause angina. This also increases the risk of an artery becoming blocked by a blood clot, causing a heart attack or stroke.

On the other hand, your body also produces high density lipoproteins (HDLs, "good" cholesterol) which are quickly transported from the bloodstream and do not as readily form atheroma deposits in the arteries.

TRIGLYCERIDES

What many people don't realize, however, is that triglycerides, a type of fat, are also now thought to be associated with increased risk for heart disease.

Previously major changeable risk factors for heart attack included smoking, high blood cholesterol, high blood pressure and physical inactivity. According to a study published in *Circulation*, however, high blood levels of the fat triglyceride may need to be added to the list.[7] Elevated triglycerides may be a consequence of other diseases, such as diabetes. Like cholesterol, triglyceride levels can be detected with a blood test.

Researchers say that in middle-aged and older white men, a high level of triglycerides—the chemical form in which most fat exists in food as well as in the body—may mean a higher risk for heart attack. Therefore, the scientists say, high blood levels of triglycerides should be considered an independent risk factor for heart attack. In the study, men with the highest levels of triglycerides were more than twice as likely to have a heart attack when compared to those with the lowest triglyceride levels.

"So far our study appears to provide the strongest evidence that higher triglyceride levels are related to increased risk of ischemic heart disease in men independent of other major risk factors such as total cholesterol and HDL (high-density lipoprotein) cholesterol," says Jørgen Jeppesen, M.D., of the Epidemiological Research Unit, Copenhagen University Hospital, Denmark.

In a recent editorial, former American Heart Association President Antonio Gotto, M.D., said that while additional research is necessary to determine whether lowering triglyceride levels can reduce heart attack deaths, the findings make a compelling argument for measuring triglyceride levels as part of an evaluation to determine an individual's risk for heart disease.

"The growing attention to high levels of triglycerides and increased coronary heart disease risk is encouraging to veterans of the 'triglyceride wars,'" said Gotto, dean of the Cornell University Medical School, New York City. "It's also in agreement with another trend in heart attack risk management, namely, the concept of global risk assessment."

Triglycerides are the form in which fat exists in meats, cheese, fish, nuts, vegetable oils, and the greasy layer on the surface of soup stocks or in a pan in which bacon has been fried. In a healthy person, triglycerides and other fatty substances are normally moved into the liver and into storage cells to provide energy for later use. But if liver function is impaired, then triglycerides will accumulate in the blood. Fortunately, artichoke extract supports healthy liver function.

High levels of triglycerides can influence the size, density distribution and composition of low-density lipoprotein cholesterol leading to smaller, denser LDL particles, which are more likely to promote the obstructions in the blood vessels that trigger heart attack. An excess amount of triglycerides in blood is called hypertriglyceridemia.

CHOLESTEROL-LOWERING DRUG COMPLICATIONS

The pharmaceutical industry has developed many powerful medical drugs to help people lower cholesterol levels. But there are two areas of concern. First, while we know that these drugs do lower cholesterol, the jury is still out whether they extend the life span of people with high cholesterol levels. Some studies have shown that people taking cholesterol-lowering drugs are at slightly higher risk of death than people not taking any cholesterol-lowering drugs. That is probably because these drugs tend to bind or inhibit the production of other essential nutrients necessary for heart health, or they have an adverse effect on brain neurotransmitters. More recently, encouraging results have been seen from clinical trials, and we are gaining greater faith in these drugs' ability to extend healthy life span.

Quick Triglyceride Primer

Traditionally, people with less than 200 milligrams of triglycerides per deciliter (mg/dl) of blood are considered to have normal triglyceride levels. Between 200 and 400 mg/dl is borderline high; between 400 and 1,000 mg/dl is a high triglyceride level; and greater than 1,000 mg/dl is considered very high triglycerides. However, the normal range may require revision.

"A very interesting finding in our study was that people with triglyceride levels as low as 142 mg/dl were clearly at a higher risk of heart disease," says Jeppesen of the study published in *Circulation*. "We believe this is of substantial clinical interest since a triglyceride level of below 200 mg/dl is usually considered 'safe.'"

In the study of 2,906 white men who were initially free of any heart disease, researchers found that during an eight-year follow-up period, 229 men had a heart attack. By examining this group of men, the scientists found that heart attack risk increased in those with the highest levels of fasting triglycerides (measurements taken after 12 hours of fasting prior to the test).

"When the triglyceride levels were measured by the amounts of HDL cholesterol in the blood, a clearer picture emerged," says Jeppesen. "Even those who had high HDL levels, which are thought to protect against heart attack, were still found to be at higher risk for heart disease because of their triglyceride levels."

The American Heart Association says that changes in lifestyle and dietary habits—cutting down on calories, reducing saturated fat and cholesterol in the diet, reduced alcohol intake and a regular exercise program—can help in the treatment of hypertriglyceridemia. Perhaps, however, the AHA should add to this list using artichoke extract daily.

Another area of concern is increased cancer risk. An industry-funded study of pravastatin (Pravachol) reported a rate of breast cancer twelve times higher than among women not using the drug.[8] Bristol-Myers Squibb, the drug's manufacturer, claimed this to be a "statistical fluke."[9] This finding is of particular importance in view of the growing numbers of patients being placed on this drug, one of four similar ones on the market.[10] Moreover, a recent report in the *Journal of the American Medical Association* concluded that commonly used cholesterol-lowering drugs, fibrates and statins, cause breast besides other cancers in rodents and that their use "should be avoided."[11] In life-threatening situations, medical drugs obviously have important uses. Still, in the area of preventive medicine, natural cholesterol-lowering agents are probably a wiser choice.

ARTICHOKE EXTRACT: NATURAL MEDICINE FOR LOWERING CHOLESTEROL AND TRIGLYCERIDES

Fortunately, nature's own pharmacy offers a wide range of safe and effective agents for reducing cholesterol. A dietary supplement program that includes a wide range of these natural cholesterol-lowering agents may not only be equally effective, it may also be much safer for consumers. Artichoke extract is one such natural medicine that is also able to lower both cholesterol and triglycerides without complications associated with medical drugs.

Artichoke leaf extract works in two ways. The ability of artichoke extract to stimulate bile flow is associated with a decrease in serum cholesterol since the bile represents a major pathway for the elimination of cholesterol (both in free form and after conversion to bile acids) from the human body. Artichoke extract also appears to inactivate or inhibit the enzyme responsible for cholesterol production.

SCIENTIFIC AND MEDICAL EVIDENCE

We know that artichoke extract is very effective at lowering cholesterol levels from a variety of types of studies, including those done in the test tube (*in vitro*), as well as other experimental and clinical studies.

Test Tube and Experimental Studies

◆ High-dose aqueous extracts from artichoke leaves were found to inhibit cholesterol biosynthesis in experimental studies.[12] The results demonstrated that artichoke extracts may inhibit hepatic cholesterol biosynthesis in an indirect but efficient manner.

◆ In the test tube, when liver cell cultures have been incubated with artichoke extract they have shown a significant inhibition of cholesterol biosynthesis within two hours.[13]

Clinical Studies

◆ As early as 1957, a decrease in serum cholesterol and phospholipids was noted in an open clinical trial involving 83 patients.[14]

◆ In 1959, researchers also reported artichoke extracts could decrease serum cholesterol.[15]

◆ In 1973, researchers found that using only 60 mg of artichoke leaf extract daily produced a 31 percent decrease in serum cholesterol and 82 percent decrease in triglycerides among 132 patients.[16]

◆ In 1974, a small study of 20 patients showed significant decreases in serum lipids.[17]

◆ In 1975, researchers reported decreased cholesterol and pre-beta-lipoproteins among 60 patients.[18]

◆ In 1979, 17 patients taking artichoke extract for only four weeks experienced a significant 15 percent decrease of serum cholesterol.[19]

◆ In a study involving 553 patients whose average age was 54.7 years, it was found that on average the patients using artichoke extract for fewer than six weeks experienced significant declines in total cholesterol and triglycerides; total cholesterol decreased from 264.24 mg/dl to 233.91 mg/dl for an average decrease of 11.48 percent. Serum triglyceride levels decreased from an average of 214.97 mg/dl to 188.07 mg/dl for an average decrease of 12.51 percent. There was also a slight increase in beneficial HDLs from 49.10 mg/dl to 52.91 mg/dl.[20]

THE BOTTOM LINE

Artichoke extract is an extremely safe cholesterol- and triglyceride-lowering agent whose greatest benefits will appear among persons with the highest levels of cholesterol and triglycerides. You can expect typical cholesterol and triglyceride reductions of 10 to 70 percent respectively when you use artichoke extract.

It is true that some cholesterol-lowering drugs may be more powerful, but we believe that artichoke extract is a safer alternative for many persons, especially when combined with a low-fat diet and additional dietary supplements noted for lowering cholesterol and triglycerides such as inositol hexaniacinate and fresh garlic products (see page 38 for information on how to obtain these formulas). You may also want to consider adding a fiber supplement and tofu to your diet. Both also have a beneficial impact on lowering blood lipids.

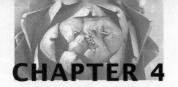

CHAPTER 4

Artichoke Extract
and Liver Protection

Do you work in an occupation where you are exposed to toxic chemicals? Are you a moderate to heavy consumer of alcohol? Do you live in a polluted area? Have you ever suffered from hepatitis or other liver disorders? If you answered yes to any of these questions, your liver may be suffering damage. You will want to start incorporating artichoke extract into your daily health regimen.

Your liver is one of the most remarkable organs in the body. The liver is responsible for many functions. The liver helps to detoxify chemicals in the body including toxic chemicals such as industrial chemicals and pesticides to which we may be exposed both occupationally and from the environment or from consumer products or foods and beverages. The liver also regulates the body's blood sugar levels by storing and releasing glucose. The liver plays an important role in your body's cholesterol levels, too. The liver has considerable responsibilities in maintaining the health of the human body. It produces bile for the breakdown of food and transport of cholesterol and fats, and breaks down excess hormones like cholesterol and estrogen. It also metabolizes proteins, fats and carbohydrates.

One of the liver's responsibilities is metabolism and neutralization of many toxic compounds which could potentially cause catastrophic damage to our bodies.

Many of these compounds (oxidized fats, pesticides, industrial chemicals, artificial preservatives and flavors) are routinely ingested with our food and in detoxification put the liver's cells at a particular risk of damage or destruction.

Because the liver plays such a vital role in maintaining health and is continuously exposed to noxious compounds, its protection is vital for the achievement of optimal health. However, the liver can become damaged from exposure to environmental toxins and abuse of alcohol, common medications such as acetaminophen, and viruses and bacteria.

Impairment of bile flow within the liver can be caused by a variety of agents and conditions (see page 14), reports our colleague Michael Murray, N.D. These conditions are often associated with alterations of liver function in laboratory tests (serum bilirubin, alkaline phosphatase, SGOT, LDH, GGTP) signifying cellular damage.

However, relying on these tests alone to evaluate liver function is not adequate, since, in the initial or subclinical stages of many problems with liver function, laboratory values remain normal, adds Dr. Murray.

Among the symptoms people with liver damage may complain of are fatigue, general malaise, digestive disturbances, allergies and chemical sensitivities, premenstrual syndrome, and constipation. Artichoke extract may ultimately be shown to be helpful in all of these conditions, thanks to its beneficial impact on liver function.

Perhaps the most common cause of cholestasis and impaired liver function is alcohol ingestion. In some especially sensitive individuals, as little as one ounce of alcohol can produce damage to the liver, which results in fat being deposited within the liver. All active alcoholics demonstrate fatty infiltration of the liver.

The pharmacology of artichoke extract centers around its beneficial effects on the liver. First of all, artichoke extract has been shown to enhance detoxification reactions as well as protect the liver from damage. This combination of effects is very important to healthy liver function. During detoxification in the liver, the toxic substance is often initially converted to an even more toxic form. Without adequate protection, every time the liver neutralizes a toxin, it is damaged in this process. Artichoke extract has been shown to provide this valuable protection.

Once the liver has modified a chemical toxin, it needs to be eliminated from the body as soon as possible. One of the primary routes of elimination is through the bile. However, when the manufacture of bile is reduced or the secretion of bile is inhibited, such toxins stay in the liver and body longer. Once again, artichoke extract can help.

Studies show the excellent detoxification results can be expected by using artichoke extract daily alone or in combination with other liver-protective herbs such as milk thistle, licorice and dandelion root.

♦ In one experimental study, liver cell cultures were exposed to toxins such as tert-butylhydroperoxide (t-BHP) or cumene hydroperoxide. These were used to assess the antioxidative and protective potential of water-soluble extracts of artichoke leaves.[21] Both toxins stimulated the production of other chemical toxins including malondialdehyde (MDA), particularly when the cells were pretreated with diethylmaleate in order to diminish the level of the important cellular antioxidant, glutathione. The addition of artichoke extracts did not affect basal MDA production, but prevented the toxin-induced increase of MDA formation in a concentration-dependent manner when presented simultaneously or prior to the peroxides. The protective potential closely paralleled the reduction in MDA production and largely prevented liver cell death (necrosis) induced by the toxin's by-products. The artichoke extracts did not affect the cellular level of glutathione, but diminished the loss of total glutathione and the cellular leakage of this important antioxidant, resulting from exposure to t-BHP. Chlorogenic acid and cynarin accounted for only part of the antioxidative principle of the extract which was resistant against tryptic digestion, boiling, acidification, and other treatments, but was slightly sensitive to alkalinization. These results demonstrate that artichoke extracts have a marked antioxidative and protective potential for the liver.

◆ Another study tested artichoke extract for its influence on sympatho-adrenal system (SAS) activity in experimental inhalation exposure to carbon disulfide.[22] Activity of SAS was assessed through excretion of noradrenalin and adrenalin. Findings indicated the SAS response depended on the concentration and duration of carbon disulfide exposure. With exposure to smaller amounts of carbon disulfide, SAS activity was observed to decrease in the second month, followed by increases in the fourth and sixth months. With exposure to much higher dosages, SAS activity was elevated over the whole period of study. Under the influence of the artichoke preparation, catecholamines, increased by carbon disulfide exposure, returned to normal. This trend was more marked for noradrenalin.

◆ There's more clinical evidence. In a human study, 62 men producing artificial fibers in a toxic work environment were administered artichoke extract as a preventive for two years.[23] Spontaneous and ADP-induced platelets aggregation was examined, since the toxic chemicals to which they were exposed caused platelet aggregation, which can lead to circulatory disease. The platelets' ability to aggregate, whether spontaneously or by induction, was found to be significantly reduced. The spontaneous aggregation after two years of administration was reduced on average by 51 percent.

BOTTOM LINE

As with other natural medicines, artichoke extract's benefits are multi-faceted. Not only is it excellent for overcoming digestive and cholesterol and triglyceride problems; it also can be extremely helpful in maintaining healthy liver function in a toxic world. Anyone working at a job with potentially toxic exposures should be using artichoke extract, possibly combining it with a quality milk thistle formula.

Consumer Shopping Tip

In regard to a general tonic to improve liver function and detoxification, artichoke extract should be your first choice. However, in cases of viral hepatitis (acute or chronic), milk thistle may be a better choice.

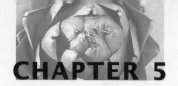

CHAPTER 5

Shopping for and Using a Quality Artichoke Extract

One of the key issues when purchasing herbs is in what form to make your purchase. Herbs are available in several different forms: bulk herbs, teas, tinctures, fluid extracts, and tablets or capsules. The type of preparation you select is a key to the results you will receive from that herb.

It is important to understand that in one form or another, most herbs are *extracted*. For example, when an herbal tea bag steeps in hot water, this is actually a type of herbal extraction process known as an *infusion*.

In this case, the solvent used to extract the medicinal substances from the herb is water. Still, although teas are a wonderful way to enjoy the mildest benefits of herbs and are certainly healthy, their ability to deliver documented medicinal benefits is limited.

An evaporated U.S. Pharmacopoeia Fluid Extract or Solid Extract is prepared by evaporation methods to remove all liquid and is concentrated at ratios of up to 50:1 or stronger. That means it would take 50 times or more of the crude herb to equal the amount in the extract. Put another way, one gram of a very typical 4:1 extract is concentrated from 4 grams of crude herb.

A solid extract is produced by further concentration of the extract, using the mechanisms described above for fluid extracts as well as other techniques such as thin-layer evaporation. The solvent is completely removed, leaving a viscous extract (soft solid extract) or a dry solid extract, depending on the plant portion or solvent used and on whether a drying process was used. The dry solid extract if not already in powdered form can be ground into coarse granules or a fine powder.

Milligram for milligram, solid extracts, sold as capsules and tablets, are the most concentrated herbal products available. In the most concentrated extracts, all excess liquid is removed through various drying procedures leaving powder. Further extractions, such as thin layer evaporation, concentrate the preparation even more.

IMPORTANCE OF STANDARDIZATION IN HERBAL MEDICINES

Due to selection of herbs, the actual strength of the active ingredients can vary. Expressing the strength of an extract by concentration still does not guarantee its potency because there may be great variation among manufacturing techniques and selection of raw materials. A standardized extract helps to provide herbs with guaranteed potency.

The term standardized extract or guaranteed potency extract refers to an extract guaranteed to contain a specific level of active compounds. Stating the content of active compounds rather than the concentration ratio allows for more accurate dosages to be made.

These types of herbal extracts represent a significantly higher standardized level of the major active constituent within the herb while still allowing for a full complement of all known and yet to be discovered active principles. Some extracts are standardized by identifying an active constituent and guaranteeing a consistent level of the constituent in the preparation. In this case, no alteration of the ratio of constituents within the plant takes place. It should be emphasized that a standardized extract provides all of the goodness of the whole plant. It is by no means a drug in the modern medical sense.

Products containing standardized extracts are guaranteed to contain a specific level of scientifically identified bioactive compounds from bottle to bottle and season to season. This allows a more precise dosage to be delivered.

This is important. Human sensitivity to an herb could vary by eight fold, notes Rob McCaleb, president of the Herb Research Foundation. "An appropriate dose of [a nonstandard-ized herb] for one person could be eight times too much for someone else," he says. "Thus, it is important [herbal] products be consistent from dose to dose."

For this reason, only standardized forms of artichoke extract should be used by health-conscious consumers. These represent the best consumer value and reliability.

HOW TO OBTAIN ARTICHOKE EXTRACT

Today, the only standardized artichoke extract available to the health food store consumer is produced by Enzymatic Therapy. One of the nation's most quality conscious and innov-ative manufacturers of natural medicines, the Enzymatic Therapy **Artichoke Extract** formula conforms to and even exceeds the standards set forth by the German Commission E, a European regulatory body recognized worldwide for its estab-lished standards for natural medicines.

Enzymatic Therapy's **Artichoke Extract** is produced at sub-stantially higher standardized levels than the extracts cited in European clinical studies—approximately five times higher, in fact.

While many German artichoke products typically contain only a 5:1 herb-extract relation (five pounds of fresh plant used to produce one pound of extract) and are standardized for only

Dosage Recommendations for Artichoke Extract

We recommend that consumers purchase an artichoke extract standardized to contain 13-18 percent caffeoylquinic acids calculated as chlorogenic acid. Consumers should take one to two 160 mg capsules three times daily with meals.

3% caffeylquinic acids, Enzymatic Therapy's product contains a notable 23:1 ratio, and is standardized at 15% caffeylquinic acids.

To find a health food store nearest you carrying Artichoke Extract, call Enzymatic Therapy at 1-(800) 783-2286; 825 Challenger Drive, Green Bay, WI 54311; website: www.enzy.com.

SAFETY

Artichoke extract is a food-based extract with no reported toxicity.

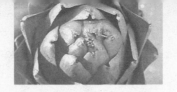

Resources

Enzymatic Therapy, a Food and Drug Administration-licensed vitamin and natural medicine manufacturer, is the first major U.S. natural medicine company to make standardized artichoke leaf extracts available in the U.S. in a supplement form in health food stores. To find a health food store nearest you carrying **Artichoke Extract**, **Gastrosoothe®** (with DGL and calcium carbonate), **Garlinase 4000®** or **Flush-Free HexaNiacin™** (for lowering cholesterol), contact Enzymatic Therapy at 1-(800) 783-2286; 825 Challenger Drive, Green Bay, WI 54311; website: www.enzy.com.

SUBSCRIBE TO
THE DOCTORS' PRESCRIPTION
FOR HEALTHY LIVING

For the latest updates on natural medicine, we recommend that you subscribe to the cutting edge publication *The Doctors' Prescription for Healthy Living* for $39.95 for 12 issues. The newsletter covers key health and nontoxic living issues monthly. Their address is 1801 Chart Trail, Topanga, CA 90290. They may be reached via E-mail at info@freedompressonline.com or visit their website at www.freedompressonline.com.

FREE to all new subscribers!

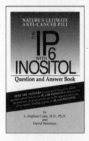

Subscribe for two years to **The Doctors'**
Prescription for Healthy Living and receive a
FREE copy of **Nature's Ultimate Anti-Cancer**
Pill: The IP$_6$ with Inositol Question and
Answer Book, the fantastic new book about the
most important natural anticancer pill of the new
millennium. Written by L. Stephen Coles, M.D.,
Ph.D., and David Steinman, this is the book that
a Congressional committee has already requested
and that you NEED to prevent and treat cancer.

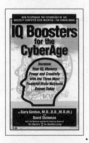

Receive two more bonuses with every two-year
subscription: *The Men's Essential Guide to Prostate
Health* and *IQ Boosters for the CyberAge*—FREE!

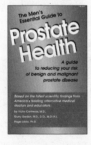

FREE to all two-year subscribers!

Subscribe for 24 information-packed
issues and receive all of these life-
saving Bonuses—FREE!

SUBSCRIBE TO
THE DOCTORS' PRESCRIPTION
FOR HEALTHY LIVING

Yes, I want to be a smart savvy shopper. Sign me up for:

_____ 12 issues of *The Doctors' Prescription for Healthy Living.* $39.95
(Receive as a bonus: *IQ Boosters for the CyberAge*)

_____ 24 issues of *The Doctors' Prescription for Healthy Living.* $49.95
(Receive three FREE bonuses: *Nature's Ultimate Anti-Cancer Pill: The IP$_6$ with Inositol Question and Answer Book, The Men's Essential Guide to Prostate Health* and *IQ Boosters for the CyberAge*)

Name (Mr., Mrs., Ms.) _____

Address _____

City _____ State _____ Zip_____

Bill My Credit Card:
☐ Mastercard   ☐ Visa   ☐ American Express   ☐ Discover

Card No. _____

Exp. Date _____X _____
                                    (Signature)

Make checks or money orders payable to Freedom Press;
mail to Freedom Press, 1801 Chart Trail, Topanga, CA 90290

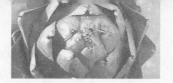

References

1   Galbraith, R.A. & Michnovicz, J.J. "The effects of cimetidine on the oxidative metabolism of estradiol." *The New England Journal of Medicine*, 1989; 321(5): 269-274.

2   Smedley, H.M. "Malignant breast change in man given two drugs associated with breast hyperplasia." *The Lancet*, 1981; 2: 638-639.

3   Kuoroda, T. & Okuda, K. "Bile acids in hepatic bile in liver disease." *Acta Hepato Gastroenterol*, 1974; 21: 120-126.

4   Held, C. "Kongreßbericht." *Therapiewoche*, 1992; 42: 1939.

5   Kirchoff, R., et al. "Increase in choleresis by means of artichoke extract. Results of a placebo-controlled double-blind study." *Zeitschrift Über Die Forschungsergebnisse Der Gesamten Medizin (Journal for Research Results From All Areas of Medicine)*, 1993; 6(40).

6   Gebhardt, R. "Antidyspeptic and lipid-lowering effects of artichoke leaf extract." *Zeitschrift für Allgemeinmedizin (Journal for General Medicine)*, 1996; 2.

7   Jeppesen, J., et al. "Triglyceride Concentration and Ischemic Heart Disease : An Eight-Year Follow-up in the Copenhagen Male Study." *Circulation*, 1998 97: 1029-1036.

8   Associated Press. "Wider use seen for drugs to reduce cholesterol of heart patients." *The New York Times*, March 27, 1996: A1.

9 *Ibid.*

10 *Ibid.*

11 Newman, T.B. & Hully, S.B. "Carcinogenicity of lipid-lowering drugs." *Journal of the American Medical Association*, 1996; 275(1): 55-60.

12 Gebhardt, R. "Inhibition of cholesterol biosynthesis in primary cultured rat hepatocytes by artichoke (Cynara scolymus L.) extracts. " *J Pharmacol Exp Ther*, 1998; 286(3):1122-8.

13 Gebhardt, E. *Medwelt.*, 1995; 46(6): 393-395.

14 Hammerl, H. & Pichler, O. *Wr. Med. Wschr.*, 1957; 107: 853-855.

15 Cima, G. et al. *Min. Med.*, 1959; 50: 2288-2291.

16 Hammerl, H., et al. *Wien. Med. Wohenschr.*, 1973; 123: 601-605.

17 Wojcicki, J. & Kadykow, M. *Pan. Med.*, 1974; 16: 127-129.

18 Montini, M., et al. *Arzneim-Forsch*, 1975; 25: 1311-1314.

19 Adam, G. & Kluthe, R. "Cholesterinsenkender effekt von cynarin." *Therapiewoche*, 1979; 29: 5637-5640.

20 Fintelmann, V. *Zeitschrift für Allgemeinmedizin (Journal for General Medicine)*, 1996; 2.

21 Gebhardt, R. "Antioxidative and protective properties of extracts from leaves of the artichoke (Cynara scolymus L.) against hydroperoxide-induced oxidative stress in cultured rat hepatocytes." *Toxicol Appl Pharmacol*, 1997; 144(2):279-86.

22 Khalkova, Z.h., Vangelova, K., Zaikov, K.h. "An experimental study of the effect of an *artichoke* preparation on the activity of the sympathetic-adrenal system in carbon disulfide exposure." *Probl Khig*, 1995; 20:162-71.

23 Woyke, M., Cwajda, H., W'ojcicki J., Ko'smider, K. "Platelet aggregation in workers chronically exposed to carbon disulfide and subjected to prophylactic treatment with Cynarex." *Med Pr*, 1981 32(4):261-4.

Special Bonus Reports

Probiotics and Gastrointestinal Health Improve Immunity

No doubt, many readers have been on antibiotic regimens, as their doctors have tried to prevent or cure secondary bacterial respiratory infections that often result when the immune system is weakened by colds or flu. Recultivating your gastrointestinal tract with friendly flora may be particularly appropriate if you have digestive problems and could also enhance your resistance to future colds or flu.

Ironically, the antibiotics that your doctor may have prescribed this winter for helping you to get through your cold or flu may end up impairing your body's immunity. That is because antibiotics have a broad-spectrum effect and destroy populations of both unfriendly and friendly bacteria.

We don't think of the friendly bacteria in our gastrointestinal tract as important components of our immune function. Yet, healthy populations of friendly bacteria play many important roles in our body's quest to defend itself against disease.

For example, take beta glucuronidase, an enzyme that disrupts our ability to detoxify environmental chemicals and hormones. High levels of beta glucuronidase in the body appear to put people at risk for breast and colon cancer.

However, a healthy flourishing population of friendly bacteria helps to displace unfriendly strains responsible for producing this enzyme. Your protection against two prevalent, often deadly cancers is thereby enhanced.

Friendly bacteria also help the body to subdue many other bacterial enemies—including *Candida albicans, Escherichia coli, Salmonella typhosa, Staphylococcus aureus* and *Streptococcus faecalis*—by acting as natural antibiotics (especially when our levels of the B vitamins folic acid and riboflavin are adequate) and by displacement as detailed above.

Besides aiding in disarming toxic chemicals, subduing unfriendly bacteria and helping the body to metabolize hormones—friendly strains of bacteria in your gastrointestinal tract help you to properly digest your food and synthesize necessary vitamins, as well as help the body to fight against yeast and urinary tract infections. So make sure your gut has a healthy population of friendly flora.

THE DOCTORS' PRESCRIPTION

If you desire maximum recolonization after using antibiotics, we recommend oral supplements containing friendly bacteria, but be extremely careful in your product selection. Poor methods of freeze drying, contamination, poor handling, variable temperatures and prolonged periods on store shelves can all contribute to highly diminished potency.

The product you purchase should be guaranteed to provide one to ten billion live strains of the two major friendly bacteria, *Lactobacillus acidophilus* and *Bifidobacterium bifidum*. (Higher amounts than this may cause gastrointestinal difficulties; smaller amounts may not provide enough live organisms for complete recolonization.)

There are a number of excellent probiotic supplements available at your health food store. The best products, such as **Enzydophilus**™ from **Enzymatic Therapy**, contain the DDS-1 strain of *Lactobacillus acidophilus*, developed by Dr. Kehm M. Shahani, professor of food science and technology at the University of Nebraska. The DDS-1 strain is far more potent than other strains and often called the "super-strain" of *Lactobacillus acidophilus*. What's more two capsules of **Enzydophilus** provide 2.5 billion bacteria that are guaranteed to be alive when they reach your gastrointestinal tract. This formula also provides fructooligosaccharides, a food that feeds friendly bacteria, and that also contributes to improved liver function, reduced cholesterol and blood pressure, and better detoxification of environmental toxins; purified colostrum from bovine sources for further immune support; and the enzymes protease, amylase and lipase for digesting proteins, fats, and starches.

Initially, take one capsule of **Enzydophilus** three times daily with meals for the first week and one capsule daily with a meal thereafter.

We recommend that anyone on antibiotics also take **Enzydophilus** concurrently to maintain the health of their gastrointestinal ecosystem. In this case, take two **Enzydophilus** capsules three times daily with meals while you are taking antibiotics and continue with one capsule three times daily with meals for several weeks following your last course of medication, reducing to the minimum dosage of one capsule with a meal about three weeks following your last use. To obtain this formula, contact Enzymatic Therapy; see our resource information on page 38.

Healing Ulcers Naturally with DGL

Sometimes indigestion is the result of an ulcer. Virtually every complementary medical doctor and naturopath agrees that the an important natural remedy for ulcers is deglycyrrhizinated licorice (DGL).

One major issue, though, for the medical consumer is what works better: mainstream medicine with its Flagyl and Tagamet or alternative medicine with its licorice? Several studies, in fact, have looked at DGL compared with Zantac or Tagamet and have shown that alternative methods work as well or better than these mainstream drugs. For example, researchers reported in 1982 in *Gut* that DGL is as effective as Tagamet for curing gastric ulcer. That same year, *Lancet* reported DGL to be as effective as Zantac, and in 1972 researchers in *Clinical Trials Journal* found DGL to be more effective than antacids. Additional supportive studies have been published in *Practitioner* and the *Irish Medical Journal*.

"The use of deglycyrrhizinated licorice (DGL) compared to standard drug therapy is a classic example of addressing the underlying cause of a condition rather than simply blocking an effect," says naturopath Michael Murray. "Most people do not get ulcers because of oversecretion of acid; the cause in most cases is a breakdown in the integrity of the intestinal lining.

PEPTIC ULCER

Peptic ulcers usually occur in the lower esophagus, stomach, duodenum, or occasionally in the small intestine. Ulcers are usually accompanied by significant damage to the mucous membranes of the gastrointestinal tract. Nutritional aids, such as a special form of licorice extract known as DGL, fresh cabbage juice and high fiber foods, are extremely helpful in healing ulcers, and aid in the eradication of *H. pylori*, the bacteria thought to play a key role in ulcer formation.

Esophageal ulcer

Stomach

Gastric ulcer

Duodenal ulcer

Duodenum

While drugs like Zantac and Tagamet can block symptoms and promote temporary healing, they do not address the underlying cause and their effects are short-lived. In contrast, DGL addresses the underlying factors and promotes true healing [by stimulating] the normal defense mechanisms that prevent ulcer formation. Specifically, DGL improves both the quality and quantity of the protective substances that line the intestinal tract; increases the life span of the intestinal cell; and improves blood supply to the intestinal lining."

The Doctors' Prescription

The DGL you choose should be supplied in chewable tablets, as many studies show this form to be most effective. When DGL mixes with saliva, this promotes release of salivary compounds, such as urogastrone or epithelial cell growth factors, which stimulate the growth and regeneration of stomach and intestinal cells, thereby protecting the stomach lining against the formation of ulcers.

Our recommended DGL formula conforms to these standards (see page 38 for information how to obtain this formula). Chew two 380 milligram tablets three times daily 20 minutes before each meal. Continue use for eight to sixteen weeks, depending on your response.

Also:

♦ Drink one liter of cabbage juice daily. Cabbage juice should be made from fresh, raw green cabbage; the recommended amount is a quart a day with results to be expected in about three weeks.

♦ Eat high fiber goods. Red and white beans, corn, and unpolished rice are particularly protective against ulcers.

♦ Avoid pain relievers such as aspirin and ibuprofen, as well as alcohol, all of which are irritating to gastrointestinal lining.

♦ Reduce consumption of milk. A 1986 study in the *British Medical Journal* found that milk actually delayed the healing of ulcers. Other substances that can aggravate ulcers include beer, 7-Up, Sanka, caffeinated teas, Coca-Cola, and wine.

About the Authors

GARY S. ROSS, M.D.

Gary S. Ross, M.D. has been in private practice with an emphasis on complementary and preventive medicine for 22 years. He is a professor of clinical medicine at Meiji College of Oriental Medicine, Berkeley, California. He lectures regularly to physicians internationally. He is on the medical scientific advisory boards of several publications and is an independent consultant within the health industry. Dr. Ross is the author of *Men's Health in Action* and other audio and video programs. He received his medical degree from George Washington University School of Medicine and did residency training in internal medicine. He is recognized for his broad understanding of the practical application of the many treatment modalities used in complementary medicine today.

DAVID STEINMAN

David Steinman is a resident of Topanga, California. He is author or co-author of *Diet for a Poisoned Planet* (Crown 1990, Ballantine 1992), *The Safe Shopper's Bible* (Macmillan 1995), *Living Healthy in a Toxic World* (Perigee 1996), *The Breast Cancer Prevention Program* (Macmillan 1997), and *Arthritis: The Doctors' Cure* (Keats Publishing 1998). He is chairman of Citizens for Health and served two years on a committee of the National Academy of Sciences where he co-authored *Seafood Safety* (National Academy Press, 1991). He is publisher of *The Doctors' Prescription for Healthy Living*, *Pharmacist's Choice* and *The Doctors' Oral Enzyme Health Letter*, three of the largest, most popular health letters in the United States today. Steinman, a graduate of Columbia University and with a master's degree in journalism from the University of Oregon, is a member of the teaching faculty at National University and the University of Phoenix. He has won awards from the California Newspaper Publishers' Association, Sierra Club, and Society of Journalists' *Best of the West*. He is married to the artist Terri Steinman and they have one son.